Sentimental Journey

A Trip Down Memory Lane

Kristine Forgit

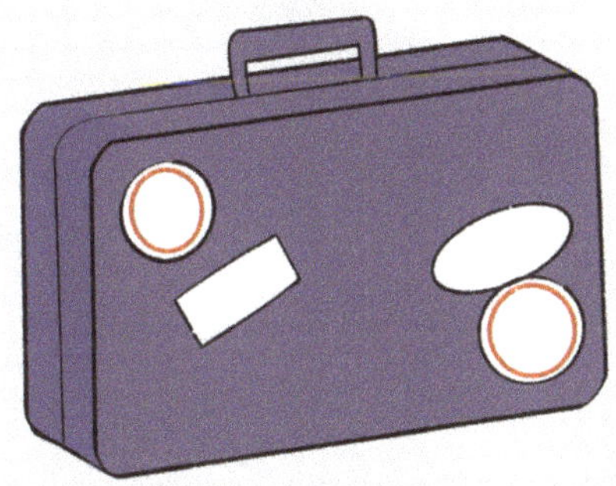

Kristine Forgit
Sentimental Journey / Kristine Forgit. —1st ed.

Paperback: 978-1-956989-37-3
Hardcover: 978-1-956989-38-0

Printed in the United States of America.

Gonna take a sentimental journey
Gonna set my heart at ease
Gonna take a sentimental journey
To renew old memories

Opening lyrics to "Sentimental Journey"
Music written by Les Brown and Ben Homer,
Lyrics written by Bud Green.

A personal memoir of "You", because you
are so special to me.

Love,

____

I will never forget when my Father first showed signs that something was changing with his ability to remember things. He was slowly forgetting how to get back home when he went for a drive, he lost his ability to concentrate and to be capable of having deeper conversations.

Dementia was taking away my Dad and our ability to travel together, go out to dinner, and have meaningful connections. I lost the Dad I knew that I could share the good and bad moments of my day, ask for advice, or have him call me just to check in on me. Over time, as he continued to decline, our times together were spent taking long rides where he would sing songs from the 1940's, his favorite music from his years of being the leader of a Classic Big Band. He would only engage in small talk if I asked him questions.

I longed to find a way to preserve our memories in the present and to provide him with the ability to remember special times such as his passions, favorite hobbies, holiday celebrations and our family. I frequently sent him cards and would write about his favorite activities, and tell him about my and my daughter's day. He read the cards aloud every day and it brought him pleasure and comfort.

That's the reason behind the creation of my book, "Sentimental Journey," a title inspired by one of my Dad's favorite 1940's songs, which he used to play on the clarinet and saxophone. This journal is designed for families to take a walk down memory lane.

My aspiration is that this book will provide you and your loved one with precious moments together, rekindling fond memories so that you too, can embark on a Sentimental Journey and hold their memories in your hand.

Wishing you a collection of cherished memories,

Kristine Forgit

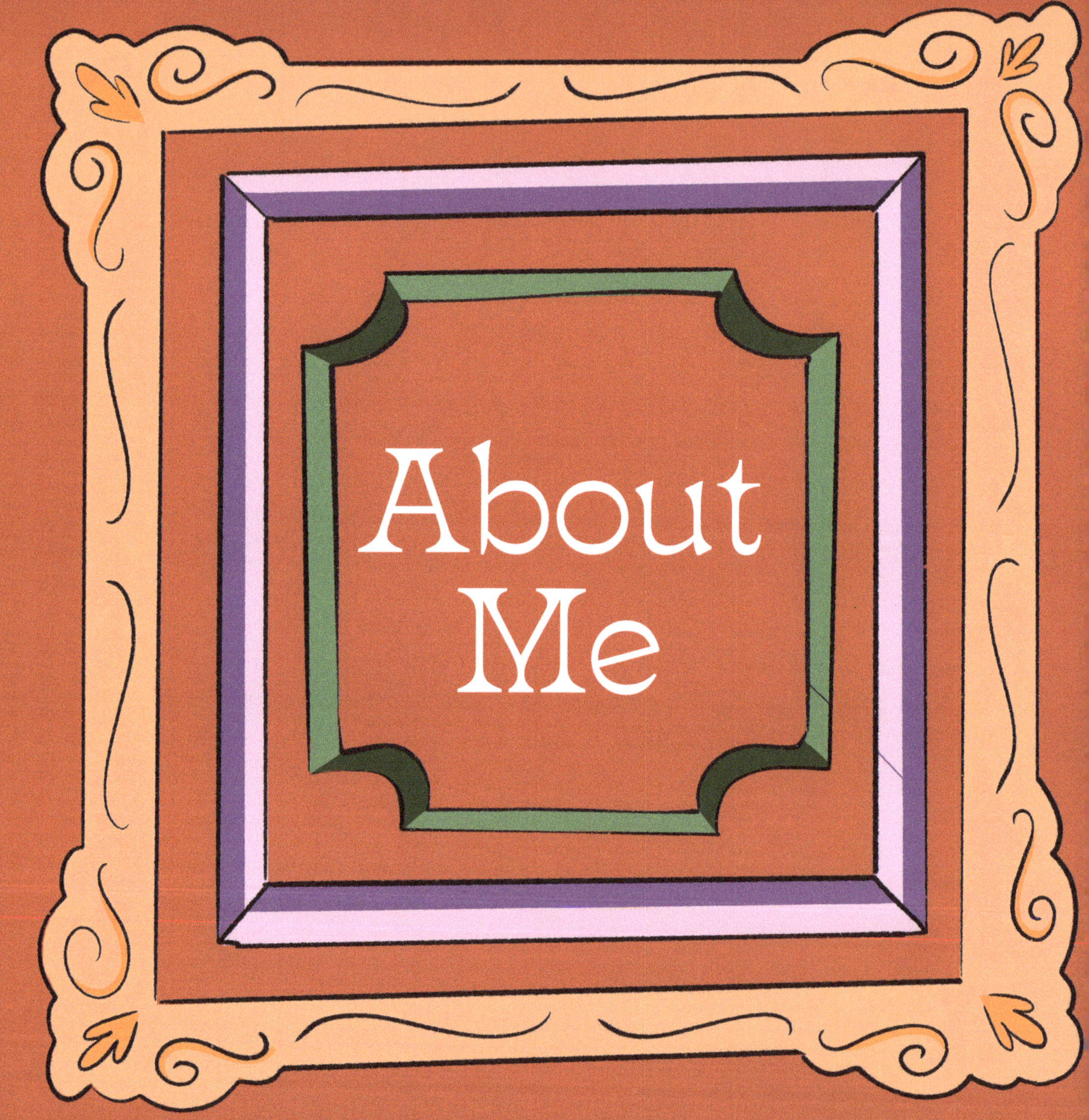
About Me

My birth name:

Now I liked to be called:

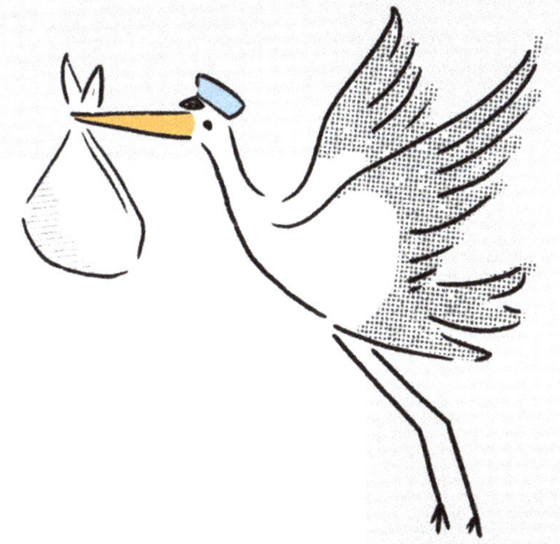

My place of birth:

____ .

I was born on ____________________________________

in the year of ________________ .

I lived in a town named

____

in the state of

______________________________ .

More about me:

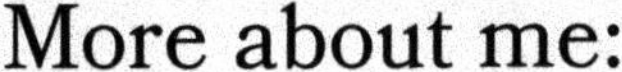

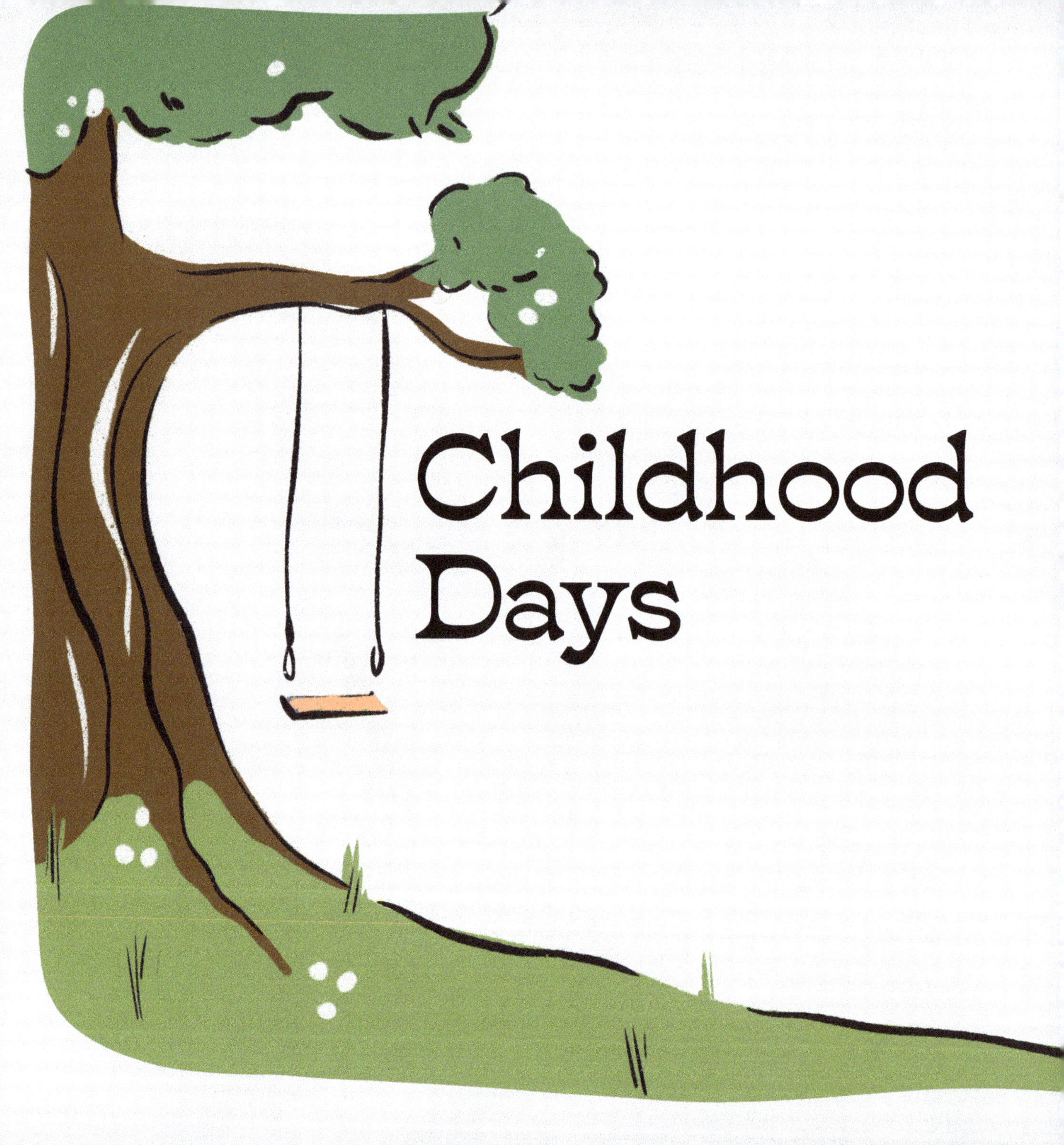

Childhood
Days

My favorite childhood memory is:

Some of my favorite places to go when I was young
were to:

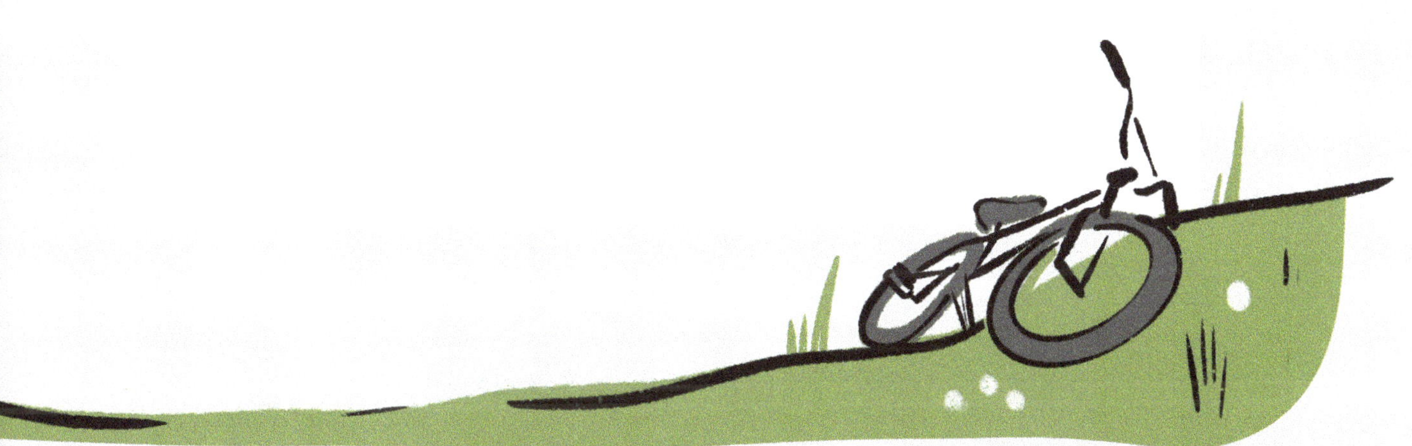

As a family, we loved to

____

____ together.

My favorite holiday as a child was

____.

My favorite activity when I was young was

____.

My favorite childhood song was

____.

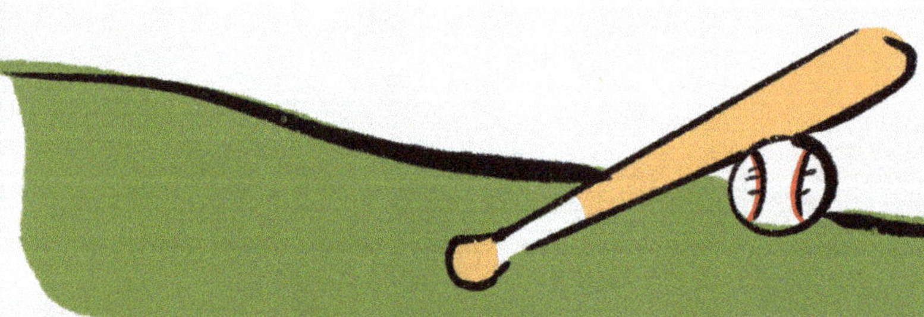

My favorite subject in school was

____ .

My favorite TV show was

____ .

More childhood memories:

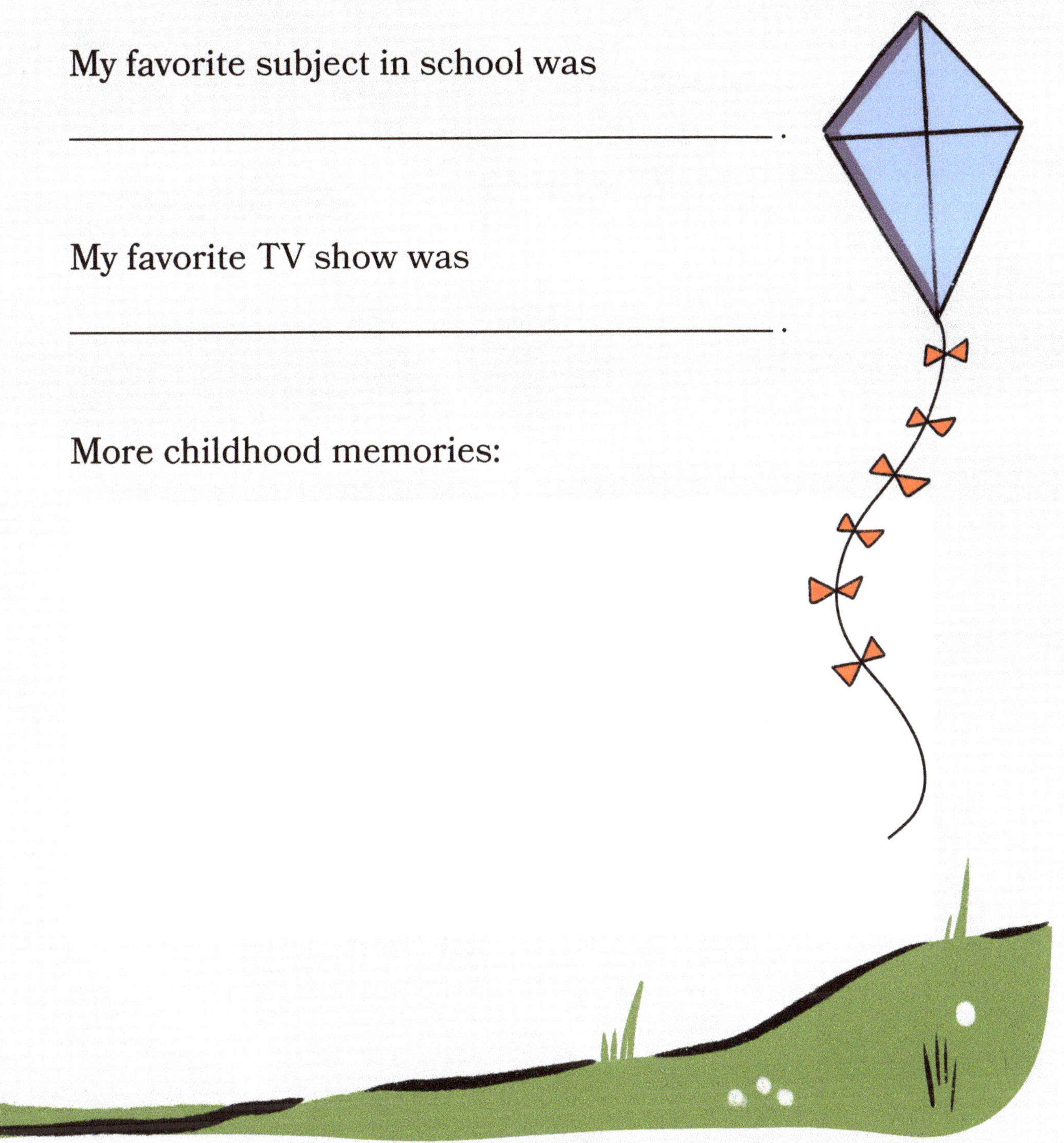

My Parents and Siblings

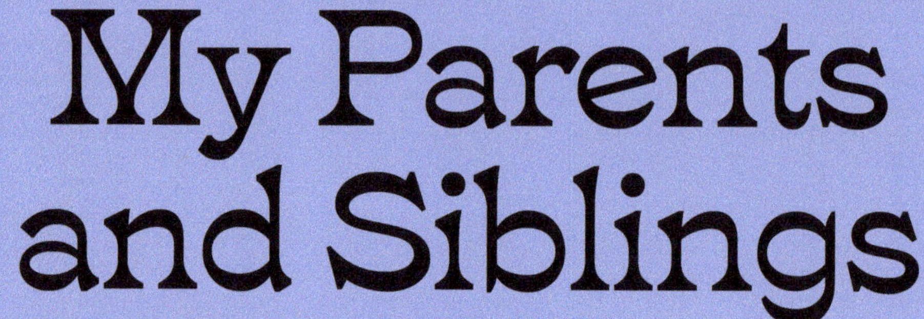

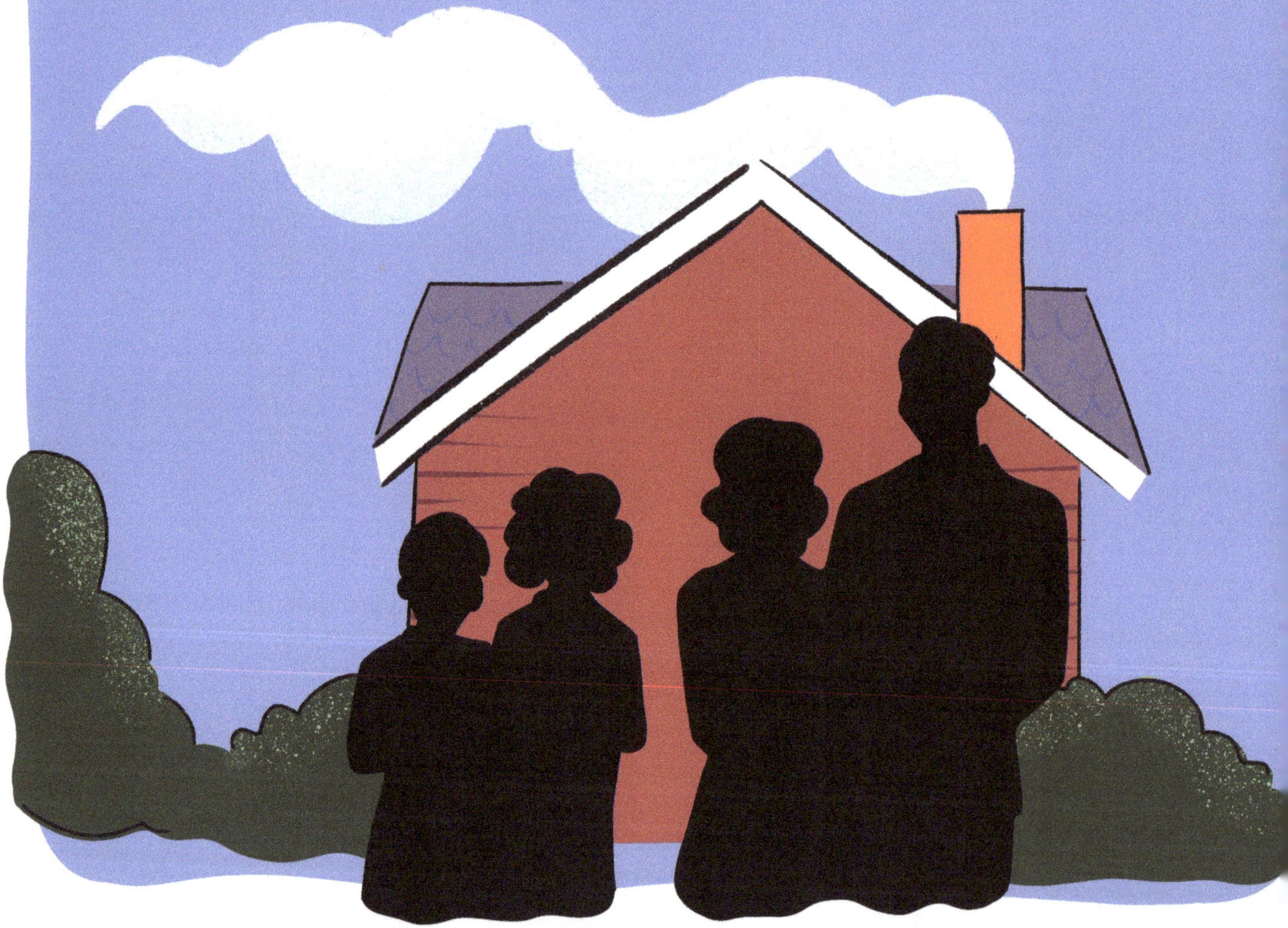

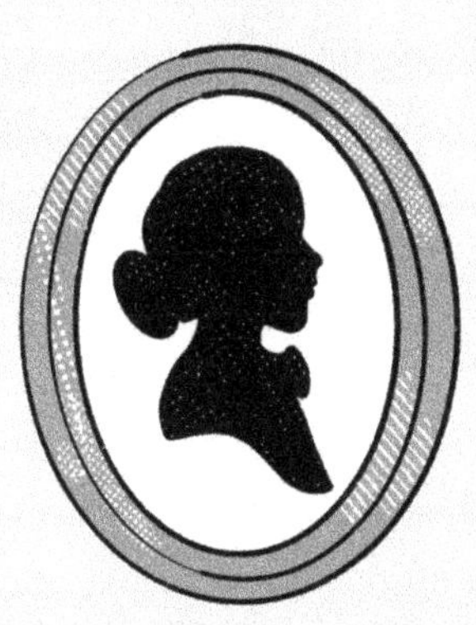

My parent's names are _________________ and
_________________.

My favorite memory of my Mom is:

My favorite memory of my Dad is:

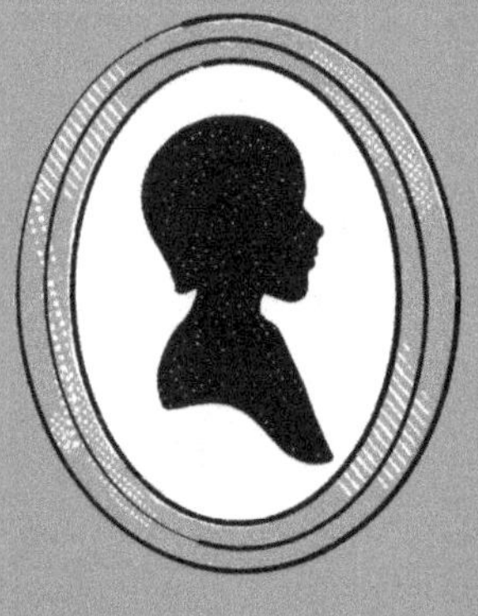

I have _________ siblings and their names are

____ .

My family always loved this about me:

____

Some of my best memories with my family is when we

____ and

____ together.

I also have extended family that includes:

____

____

____

____

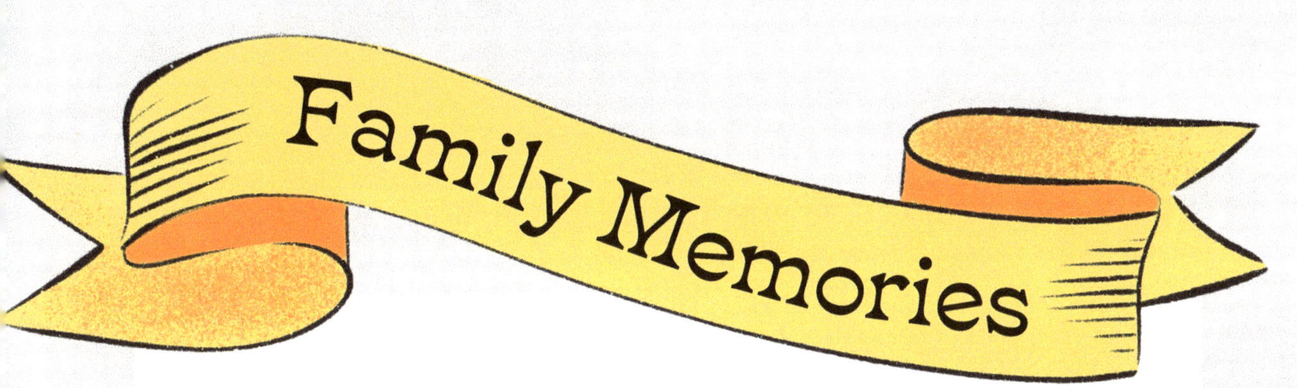
Family Memories

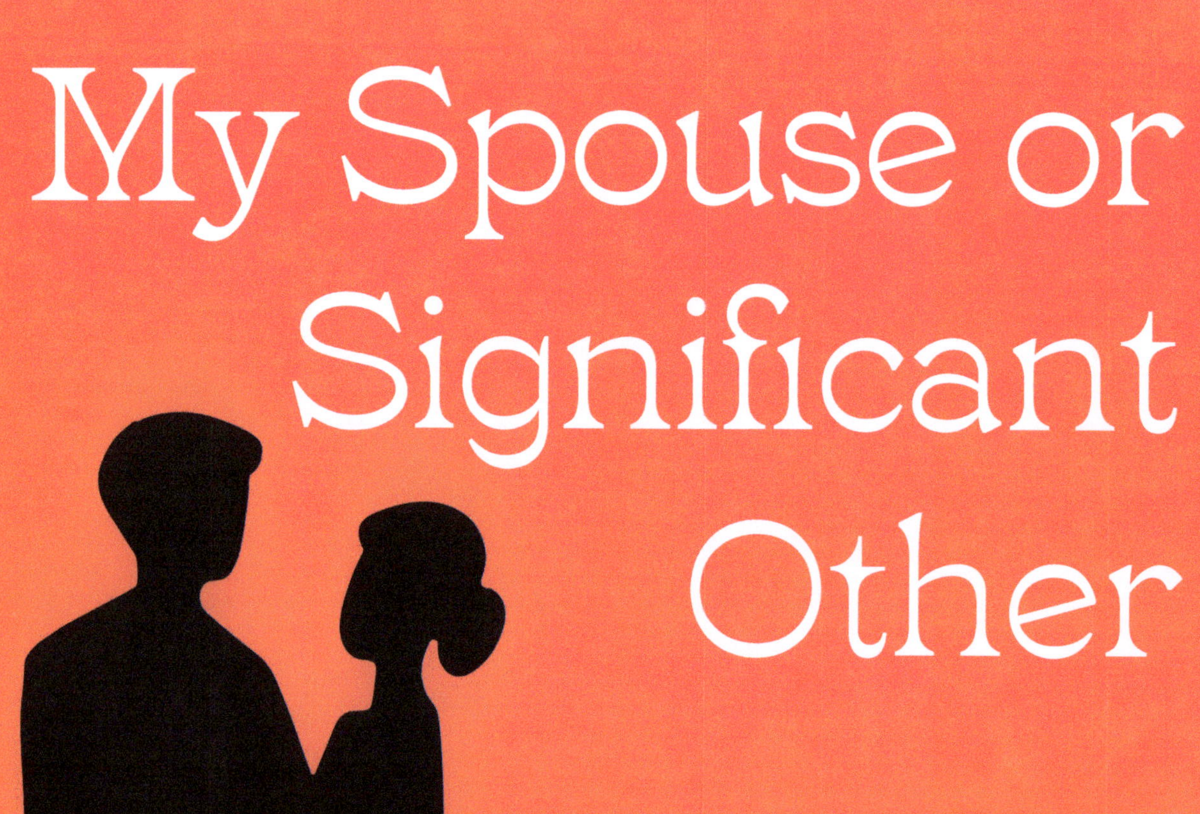

My Spouse or Significant Other

My Spouse's name:

We were married on this date:

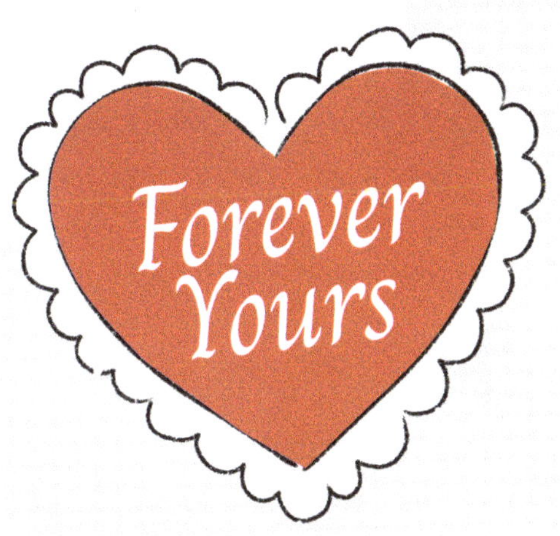

The place where we got married was

_______________________________________.

We lived in a town called

_______________________________________.

Some of my best memories together
were when we

____

____

____

____

_______________________________________.

More about my spouse/significant other:

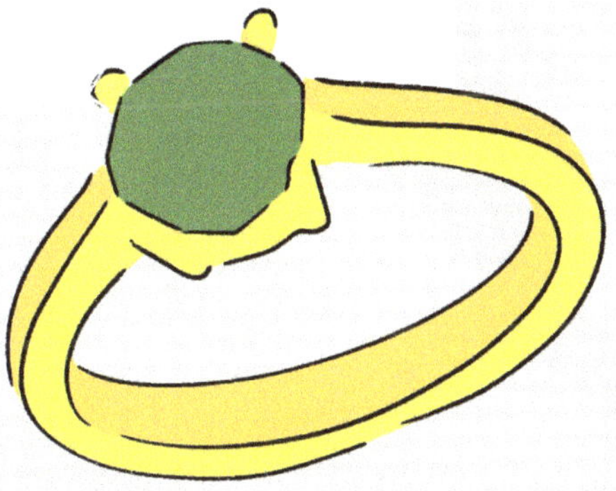

Children (and Pets)

I have _______________ children.

My children's names are:

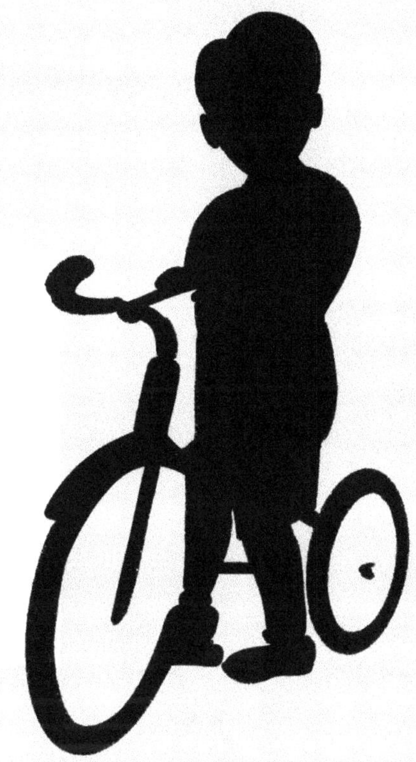

My children live in:

My favorite memory together is when we:

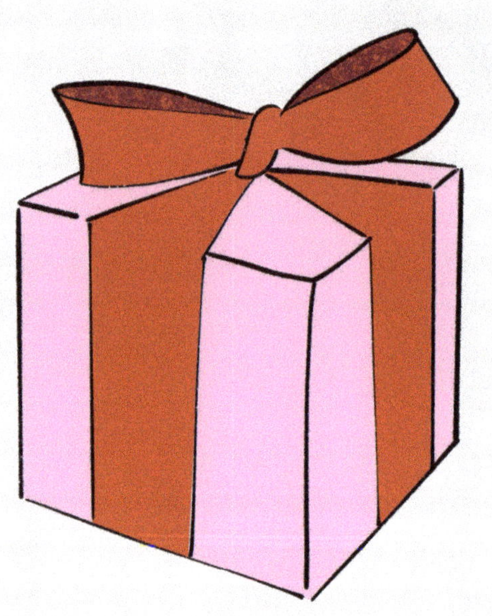

Our favorite holiday together is:

____

____

____

____

____

____

My children think I am:

More about my children and pets:

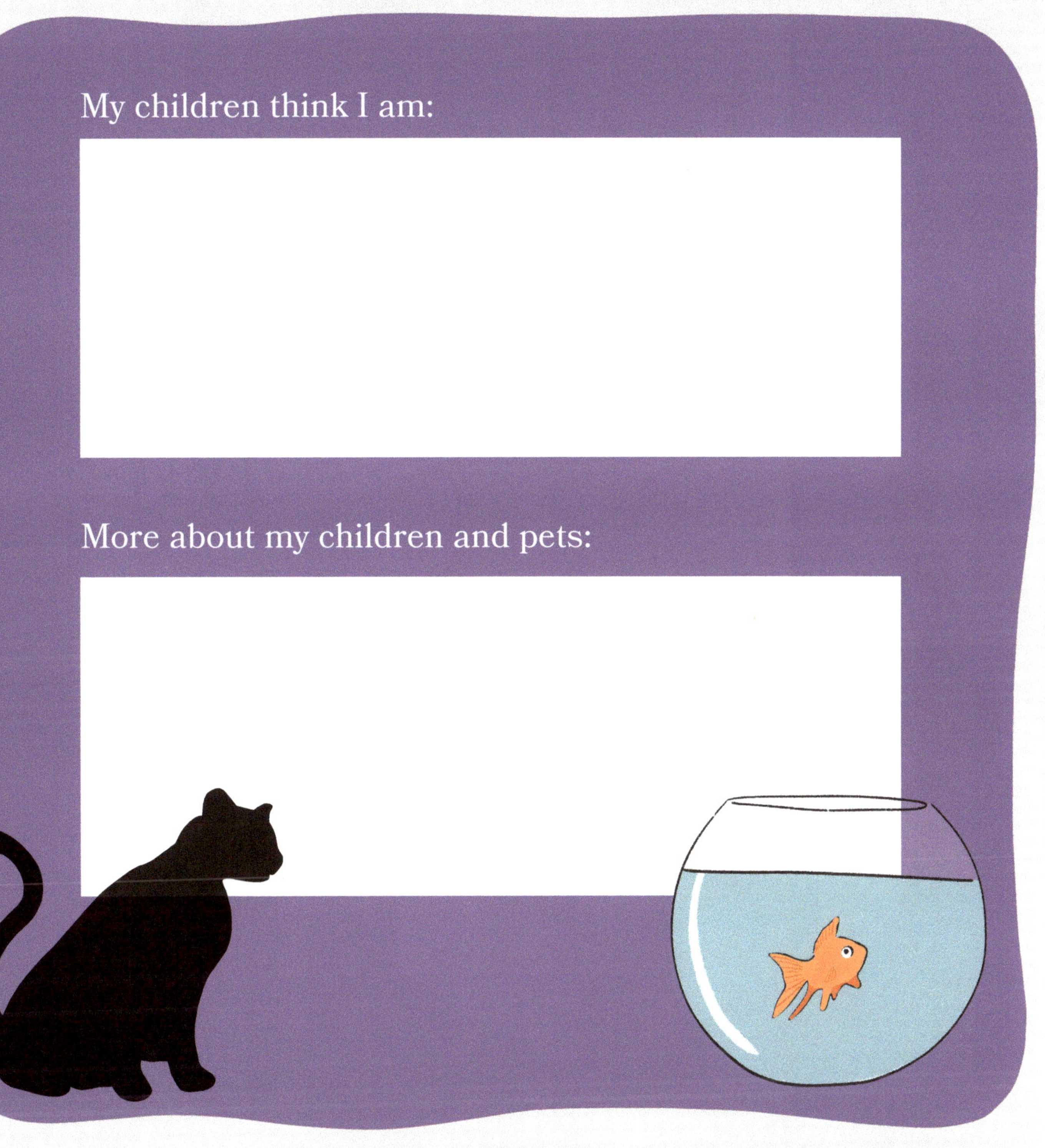

Interesting Facts About Me

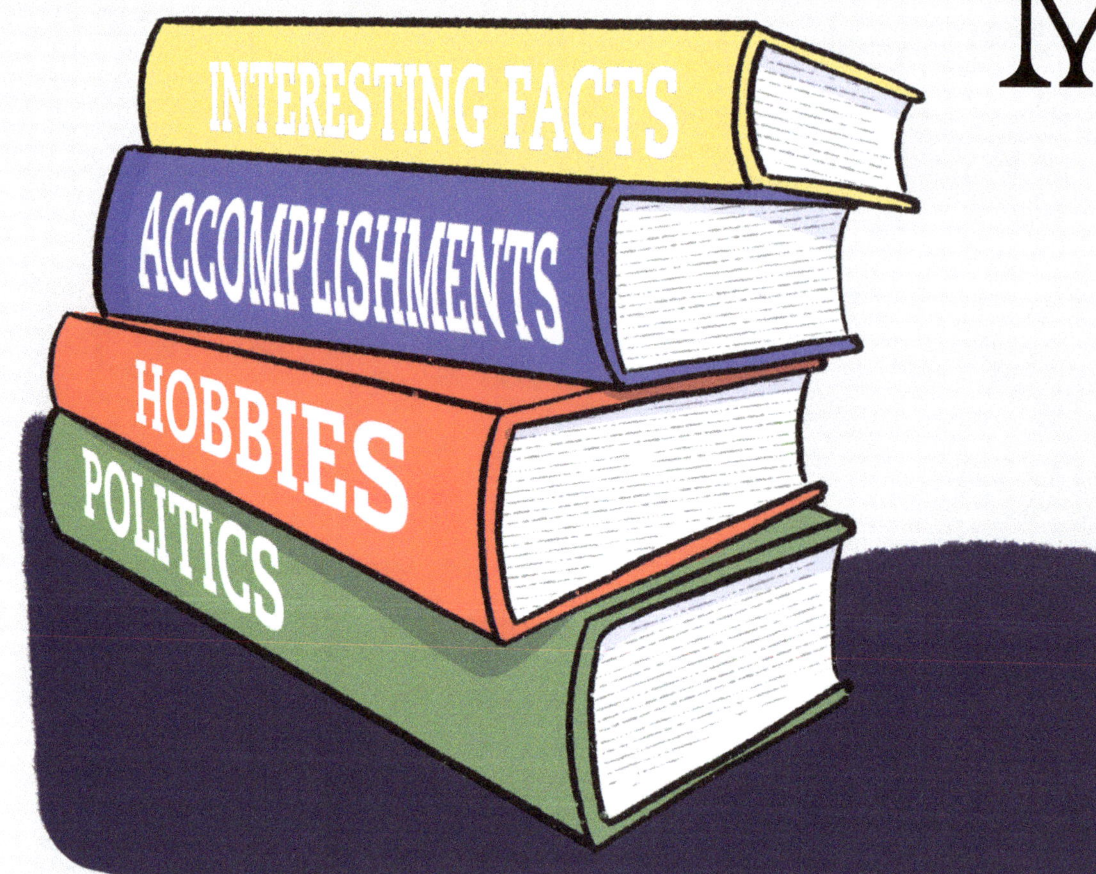

My accomplishments:

My hobbies:

My favorite activities:

My religious and political views:

My dislikes:

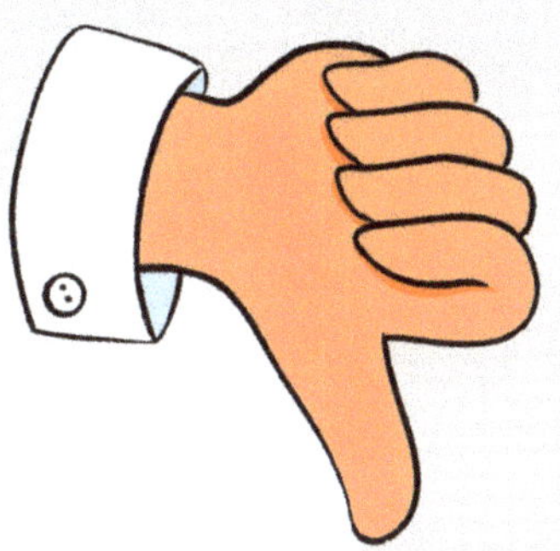

My favorite places:

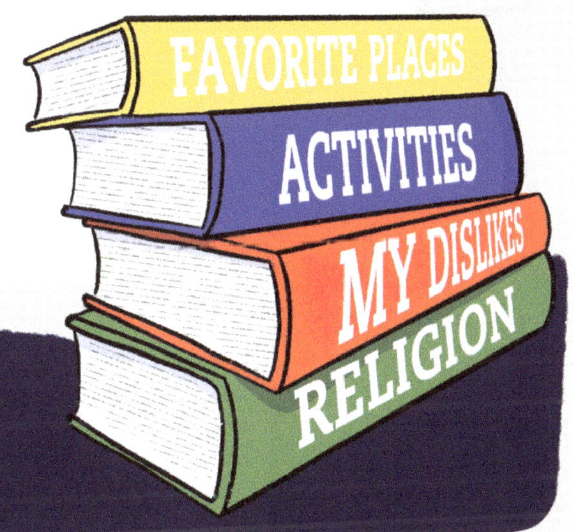

My Favorite Things

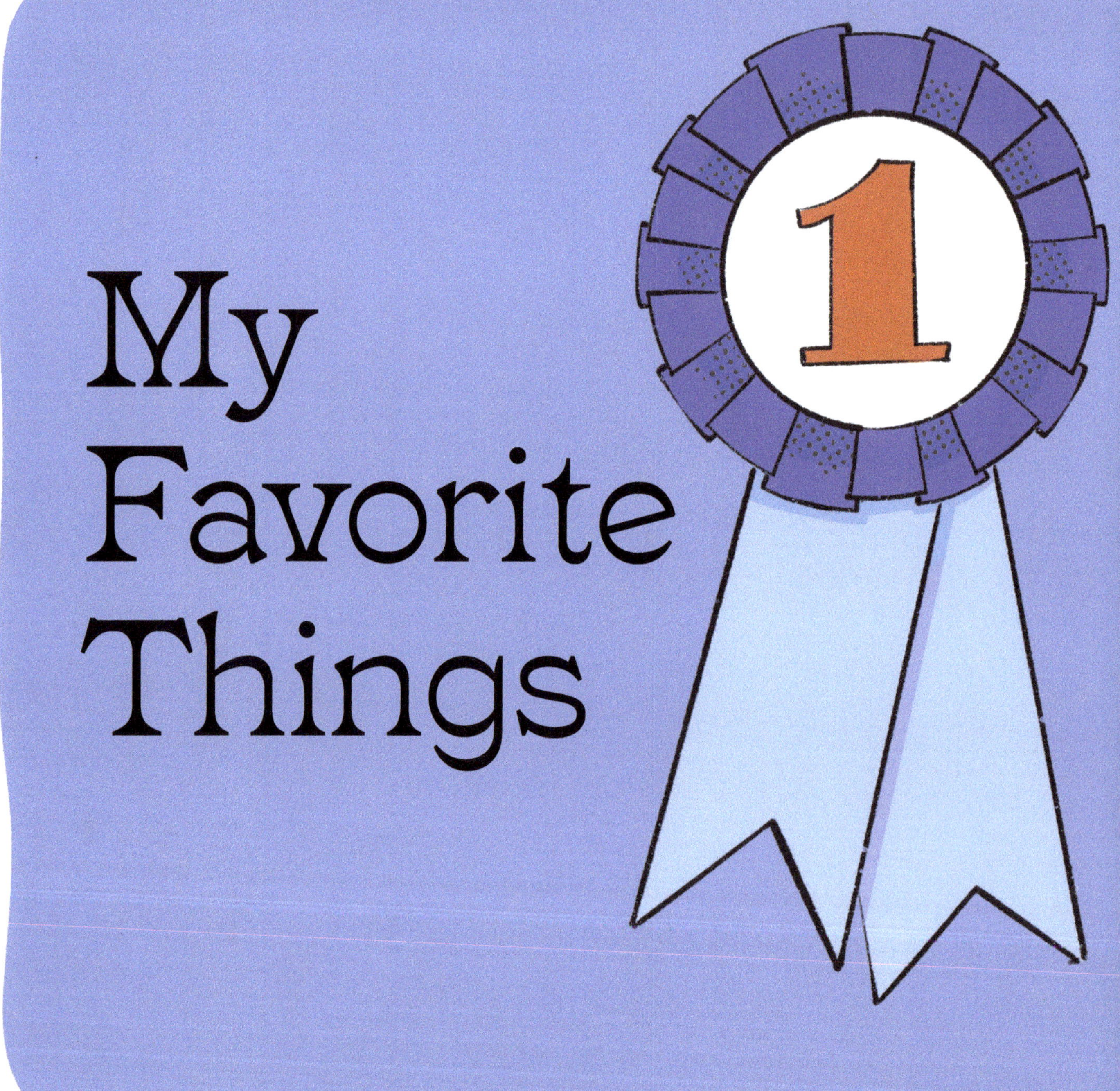

My favorite color is:

My favorite food is:

My favorite flavor of ice cream is:

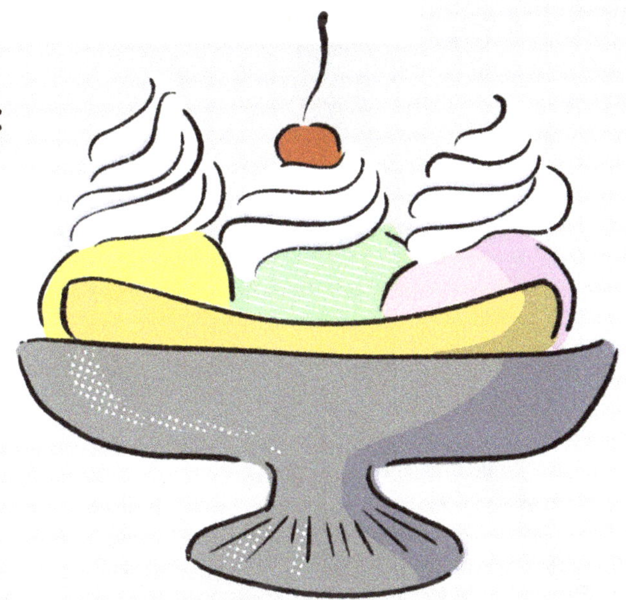

My favorite song is:

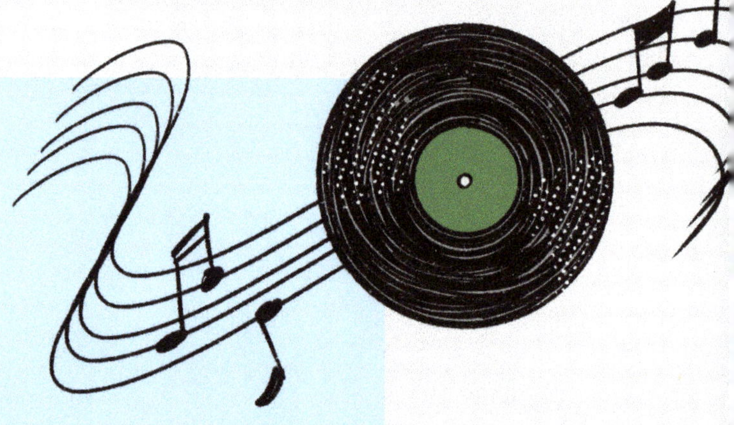

My favorite singer/band is:

My favorite sport is:

My favorite sports team is:

My favorite place to go is:

My favorite holiday is:

My favorite animal is:

My favorite season is:

____

My favorite smell is of:

____

My favorite flower is:

____

My favorite activities are:

____

____

____

____

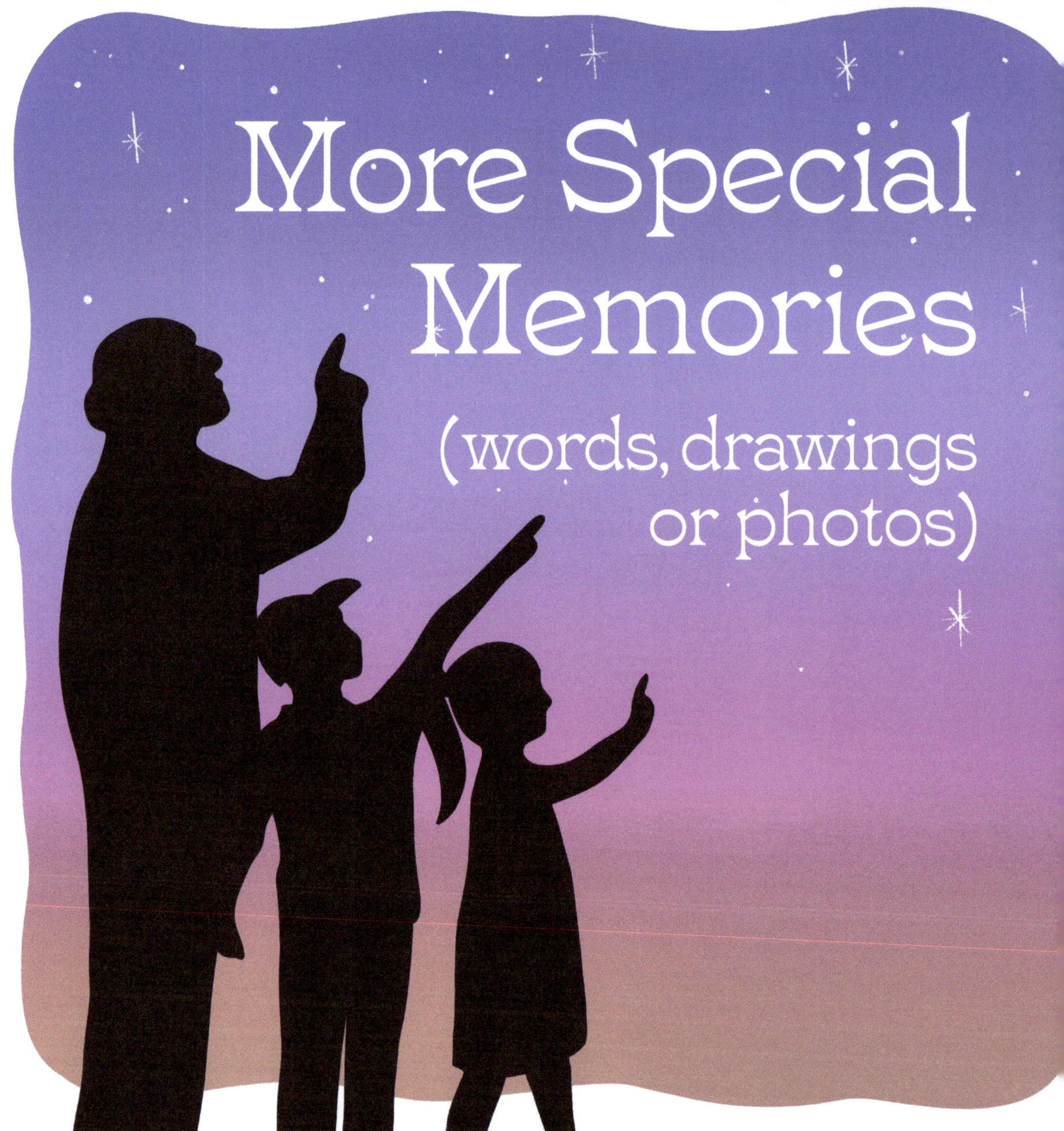

More Special
Memories
(words, drawings
or photos)